How I Turned Hurt

into Health

By

B. Blossom Lordman

ISBN-13 978-1540625717

ISBN-10 1540625710

Believe stock photo by The Path Traveler

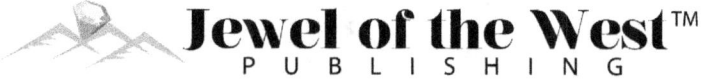

Jewel of the West™ PUBLISHING

This Book is lovingly dedicated to:

My Angel, My Grandmother

Mrs. Lucy Mae Sharp

Grandma, if I could sit and talk to you today, I know what you would say to me. You would say, "Blossom, I'm so proud of you. You have FINALLY found your voice." I miss you more and more every day. Rest in Heaven, Grandma. Save a seat for me.

To my Dear Sweet Tausha

Your beautiful life and smile was taken away from us far too soon. Cancer took your body, but your spirit will live forever! Rest in Heaven, Sweet Girl! Until we meet again.

To My Mother

Mama, we had a rough beginning, but our present, our FUTURE, is brighter than ever! I love you Mama....and together, WE HEAL and WE LIVE!

And a special thank you to author /publisher and my sister/cousin,

Jewel Adams. Without you, none of this would be possible. Thank you

for believing in me!

I love you!

Note to Reader:

Though 1 have taken pains to tone my words and

the descriptions of my experiences, my story is

raw and unapologetic, my healing ongoing.

And God is in it.

B. Blossom Lordman

Chapter 1

And So It Begins . . .

1978

Molestation is a monstrously-dirty word, and a horrendous act that no one should be subjected to.

But at five years old, molestation by a family friend altered the course of my childhood, charting my life toward a path I could never have foreseen.

James was the name of the offender, and I can still see his face and hear his voice so clearly.

He would sneak upstairs when Mama was asleep, and pick which one of us he would defile that night–me, or one of my sisters. We will call them Karen and Tina.

I always remember a red light being on with Teddy Pendergrass's slow jam, "Turn off the Lights" playing in the background–which is why I hate red lights and will not listen to that song to this day. I mean, if I am in the middle of an intimate moment and that song comes on, I will stop and change it, because I don't want to remember . . .

But how could I forget?

We never screamed and we never told, because back then, and even now in many cases, the little girl is always the one to be blamed.

"Go sit yo fast tail down somewhere!" was the response I got when I finally did tell my mother. *"You shouldn't have been fanning your behind around them grown men."*

Well, grown men should not be looking at a five-year-old like they would look at a grown woman! What about kicking the grown man out? What about locking your little girl's door at night so the sick pervert can't get in? I used to say that if I ever saw him again, I would kill him where he stood. Evidently, God had other plans because I never did.

Chapter 2

And it Continues . . .

1983

When I turned ten, it happened again, and once again everybody pointed the finger at–you guessed it–me.

I was left alone to babysit for one of Mama's friends. I was only ten, but I guess she considered me responsible enough. The brother of her friend came home. He said to let him in, and I trusted him because Mama was dating his uncle.

After being there for a bit, he asked for a hug and I gave him one. Then he asked for a kiss and I gave him one. It was the first time I had ever experienced a

French kiss. I remember not liking it, because his tongue felt like a slug. Next, he lay me down and pressed against me, trapping me between him and the couch.

I was scared and told him to stop, but he ignored me and kept going. He then unzipped his pants, and I began to freak out a little, again begging him to stop. He kept going until I finally said, "If you don't stop, I'm going to scream!"

At those words, he stopped.

Now remember, I was only ten, and even though things had not progressed past that, enough had happened that I was totally afraid I had just done something wrong! I remember we had just had a sex education class, and in my young mind, the statement that stood out most from that class was, "If you have sex, you can get pregnant!" Well, I thought what he had done to me *was* sex.

I went to the Home/School Coordinator and told her what had happened–not because I was trying to get him into trouble, but because I thought that I was going to have a baby. In my young mind, it only made sense.

Well, I guess you can imagine what happened.

Pure hell!

The counselor called the police! The police called Social Services. They in return called my Mom, and all hell broke loose!

Did Mama go after *him*? Did she chase him down with a gun or a knife for even thinking about touching her baby? Did she swear God's wrath down upon him? No! All of her anger and wrath came down on her ten-year-old daughter!

She came to the school and called me a liar, and that (here we go again) I shouldn't have had my fast tail around him. I mean she and her friend are the ones who left me with the sick jerk in the first place.

The whole ordeal was awful! A polygraph test, detectives questioning me, court dates. Ugh! I can't remember what his sentencing was, and I don't even know if he is still alive.

It was an episode filed away but never forgotten.

B. Blossom Lordman

Chapter 3

Family Connections

*T*he next abuser?

My uncle.

Yes, you read that right, my uncle. This is a man who is supposed to protect you when your parents are not around–the one who is supposed to threaten to whip your butt if he sees you acting foolish or "being fast."

My uncle was sneaky, and stealthy, touching me inappropriately here and there when no one was looking. I grew to hate him, because to me it seemed that he thought he was entitled to "sneak a feel". No remorse, no apologies, nothing!

In fact, when I was fourteen (and pregnant, which is a

story in itself) he boldly grabbed one of my breasts. I told, and of course no one believed me. However, when he tried inappropriate things with my sister Karen in his car, (I mean she literally jumped out of his moving car to get away from his advances) I thought Mama was going to die! I find it sad but funny that she never acted that way when anything happened to me. I still struggle daily with forgiving my uncle. One day I hope to hit that mark.

As I said at the beginning, molestation truly is an ugly word, one that should never be hidden. To any young girls reading this, it is NOT okay to be touched when you don't want to be. It *is* ok to say no and to mean it. Mothers, if your daughter or a younger family member comes and tells you they have been touched inappropriately, listen to them. Protect them. Please! You have no idea what disbelief can do to a young soul or the damage it can cause, and sadly, in many cases, that damage is permanent.

Chapter 4

My Mother

*I*t is hard to know where to begin when talking about Mama. First of all, let me just say that this book is not about bashing my mother. Truthfully, I love my mother with all of my heart, but my story has to be told and there is no getting around the facts. I can no longer keep hidden what should have been brought to light long ago. I can't afford to keep it bottled inside any longer. So far, it has only done me more harm than good emotionally.

Our bond should have been the closest. After all, I was the youngest, and I was born on my mother's birthday! But it was just the opposite. I love Mama, and I forgive her. But we have a rather weird relationship. I think my quirkiness got on her nerves.

Did my mother love me? I'm sure she did. Did she like me? I'm not so sure. Mama was always more concerned about my older sisters than she was about me. Sometimes I find myself wondering if that was because I had a different father.

Oh, Mama and I had our moments when we got along, but at a very young age, I was very aware of the difference in the way she treated my sisters and I.

My mother was introduced to drugs at a young age, and I often think of how my life would have been if she had not gotten addicted to drugs. I don't really blame Mama for her addiction. She was lured into it by someone who was supposed to protect her and look out for her well-being.

However, even before the drug use began, I frustrated Mama. These are the things I remember:

*She always hated doing my hair because my head was "shaped funny" according to her, but she enjoyed doing Karen and Tina's hair.

*She never allowed me to take naps with her, but when I would sneak down the hallway, I always saw

Karen not only napping with her, but sleeping on Mama's back. Again, the difference was there.

*She never believed me over Karen, no matter how mean or ugly she was to me. One thing that sticks out in my mind is mealtimes. I would finish all of my food, and then Karen would scrape her food onto my plate, claiming that she ate all of her food, and not me. No matter how much I cried or pleaded or told the truth, I was still made to eat all her food as well.

Sometimes I wonder if that's where my eating addiction came from. I often found solace at my grandparents' house; there was always an abundance of cookies, candy, and sometimes pound cake, which is still my favorite. Thinking on it further, I *know* this was the beginning of my food addiction.

Again, I'm not throwing shade on Mama, but I just realized she loved me in her own very different way.

 We moved from place to place, never really settling down too long in one spot. I don't think Mama started to abuse drugs hard until I was in the sixth or seventh grade. This is also the time she started leaving me home alone.

By this time in my life, both Karen and Tina had fallen victim to either drugs or alcohol. My oldest sister Tina had two little girls by then, and I was often left alone to care for them. There were many nights when I didn't know what I was even going to feed us.

I hated going to school, because often there were no clean clothes, and I was tired of being picked on because of it. Sometimes the only reason I even went to school was to get something to eat. But the teasing soon became too much to bear, so I started staying home.

Most times Mama, Karen, and Tina would leave Tina's kids with me, with no running water, no power, and very minimal food. Those were dark times for me. It is painful to sit here and write about it, but this is the only way I can heal.

I can remember one Christmas season when there was nothing—no tree, no presents, no Christmas carols, no lights, no water, no food, no Mama, and no sisters—it was just me. I was scared and so alone.

I knew where my biological father lived, so I decided to walk to his house. I knew he would at least give me something to eat, and I figured he would just take me to my grandparents' house afterward. I'd never really spent much time with my father. Even still, I knew he wouldn't turn me away.

I didn't live that close to my father, at least not close enough for a ten-year-old child to walk. I braved the cold (Asheville, North Carolina cold,) and crossed this huge bridge (I'm totally afraid of heights.) When I reached my father's house, I knocked on his front door, unannounced. It opened and I found myself looking into the face of his wife. Talk about awkward!

We locked eyes for a split second, and I just knew she was going to send me away. As I was preparing to turn and continue on to my grandparents', she said, "Blossom, get in here, it's cold!" She never asked where my mother was, or why I was there. She invited me in and gave me the one thing that I was hoping for: FOOD!

I can't remember if this was my first time meeting my father's other daughter, but I remember her being nice to me. Her name was Sissy. Since I'd never experience kindness from a sister before, this was an unexpected and much-needed change. Nobody made me feel out of place or ashamed. Honestly, I must have looked a mess, because Sissy called her best friend Ramona to come over and do my hair. My unkempt appearance did not reflect well on my mother at all.

I remember Christmas being so magical at my father's house. My step-mom had everything decorated so pretty. Her Christmas tree was gigantic, and was surrounded with presents. She had lights everywhere and stockings hung. It was beautiful! Even the music she had playing soothed me at the time.

My stepmother could have turned me away. She could have chosen not to take her husband's child in, but she did take me in, and I wanted to stay. I didn't ever want to go back to the sadness and neglect that I'd just walked away from. Yes, my stepmother was stern–she made me take naps and she made me have manners, but darn it, I wanted to stay!

In fact, I overheard my sister saying that she wanted to keep me. I remember being so happy that someone actually wanted me–that someone really cared. My young mind had shouted, *"Yes! Finally, a way out!"*

Surely Mama would say yes! There would be one less mouth to feed; she would have the freedom to do what she wanted, so of course she would say yes. Right?

Wrong!

When they finally took me home, Sissy walked me into the house. I remember not wanting her to go in because I didn't want her to see how we lived. When we entered, Mama was sitting at the table with candles lit and I was so embarrassed. (Remember, we didn't have any power.)

Sissy asked Mama for me. She said, "Let me have her, Linda. I'll take care of her."

"No," was Mama's answer.

She tried again. "Linda, you know I'll take care of her. Let me have her."

Again, her answer was no, and I felt like I had been punched in the stomach. I didn't want to stay there in that dark house–a house full of dark souls and dark memories. I wanted to go back with my sister, back to my stepmother, and back to my father.

I wanted to go back to the Christmas music and food, and yes, even those darned naps! I wanted to scream at Mama, *"Why? Why do you want me here when you are never here?"*

Sissy finally turned to leave, and a minute later I heard her car start. I wanted to run after the car, but I knew better. I remained quiet then went to my dark room, and there I stayed, wishing for better times.

My oldest sister, Tina, and my mother had a pretty close relationship. However, I believe it was Karen that Mama loved most–the one who shared Mama's naptimes and always got me into trouble. She had a place in Mama's heart that I just could not reach. No matter how hard I tried, no matter what I accomplished in life, I just couldn't seem to find my own spot in that special part of her heart.

Karen was able to manipulate Mama; I didn't have that skill. It seemed like everything she did was right. Even when we became adults, I still felt like I had to fight for Mama's attention, so I finally decided to stop fighting. I decided it would be best to back away and let them have their relationship. I knew that eventually

I would get to have my own relationship with my mother. I prayed for that better relationship, because I didn't want anything ever to happen to either of us and not have any closure. I *needed* that.

I did question Mama when I was an adult. I will not sit here and claim that I immediately forgave her for everything because that would be lying, and I despise liars. I felt a hatred for Mama for a very long time. I would have outbursts of anger and days of tearful emotion. I would sometimes wake up in the middle of the night crying.

I finally sought out help at the local mental health clinic. They had me on so much medication that I almost didn't know who I was at times. Let me tell you something: It is hard to *feel* like you were rejected by your mother, but I truly understand now; it was drugs that took Mama away from me.

God did answer my prayers, because now I talk to my mother every day. Not only do I talk to her, but we are closer now than we have ever been. I enjoy talking to Mama, and laughing with her. I go to her for advice, and she actually comes to *me* for advice now, which blows my mind at times. Now I have the relationship with her that I've always wanted, and because of that, I love her so much!

When I look in the mirror, I see Mama. Sometimes when I speak, I hear her voice. I see her as she would be if drugs had never entered her life. I know in my soul, that had she not been introduced to the hard life of drugs, she would have been a dynamic mother to us all!

I love you, Mama!

Chapter 5

My Grandparents:

My Angels

My grandparents played a major role in my life. When things got really bad with Mama, my grandparents stepped in and came to my rescue.

One day there was nothing in the house to eat and I was really hungry. My uncle lived a little way up the road, so I decided to go there and ask him to open up a can of cranberry sauce. (That was all I could find at the moment.) He asked if Mama was making a turkey, and I told him, "No, Sir, this is all I have to eat."

He said, "Where yo Momma at?"

My answer to him was, "I don't know."

Right then God put His hedge of protection around me. Why do I say this? Remember what I told you about my uncle in the beginning? He could have chosen this opportunity to do anything to me, but instead, he made me a peanut butter and jelly sandwich and told me to go home. Feeling grateful, I grabbed my sandwich and ran home.

The next thing I knew, there was a knock at the door. I remember being scared to open it, because I had been skipping school and I just *knew* the truant officers were coming to get me. The knock grew louder, and then I heard a voice like thunder! It was my granddaddy!

"Punkin'!" he said with a loud voice. (He was the only one who called me by that name.) "Open this door!" I ran to the door, and when I opened it, I immediately wrapped my arms around my grandfather.

"Granddaddy!" I cried. Then I looked over his shoulder and saw the most beautiful, tear-stained face– the angelic face of my grandmother. They told me to get in the car and not worry about taking anything.

The first thing my grandparents did was to take me shopping for clothes, and to get a Gheri curl, because the hair was a mess, trust me. They didn't make me go back to Mama. They kept me.

~~~

I was so used to being by myself, and Mama had never been strict, but my grandparents sure were! I wasn't used to structure and being put on a schedule. I wasn't used to that kind of discipline. Despite the love I received and the stable home life, I often threatened to run away because I didn't want to follow the rules. I didn't want to go to church, or choir practice on Saturday. Heck, I didn't even want to *join* the choir.

One thing was for sure. In my grandparents' house, there was no staying home on Sundays! We had to go to Sunday school, and then to church service. If there was church at night, we had to go then too.

My grandparents instilled a work ethic in me at a young age. While my friends were sleeping in on Saturdays or at the mall, my cousins and I were doing yard work for a lady my grandmother did housework for. We got paid five dollars each.

Once I got used to my grandparents' rules (yes, I still broke them from time to time,) things started to feel normal for me. Grandma taught me so much–how to cook, how to pray, how to care for my body. She taught me everything. I would sneak down the hallway early in the mornings and hear her praying for me. I think it was those prayers that kept me out of a lot of crap!

I started to do really well in school and I made pretty good grades. And I eventually started to enjoy going to church and singing on the choir. Shoot, there wasn't much to do at home except listen to gospel records with my grandmother. We would listen to everything from Mahalia Jackson to James Cleveland. And Grandma would sing! Oh, goodness, that woman could sing! I always sang the soprano and she sang the alto.

I can still see her now, with her cup of Sanka (truthfully, I never understood why she drank decaf coffee all the time) patting her feet to the music, and telling me to embrace my voice, to come out of my shell. I didn't really think I could sing at all, but I liked singing for her.

Through my grandmother, I learned who Jesus was. One thing she definitely did was to make sure I knew him for myself. She would often say, "Blossom, don't rely on what the preacher says. Read the Bible and learn it for yourself."

Grandma and I shared some deep conversations. I won't go into what we discussed, because I always promised to keep her secrets, and she promised to keep mine.

My grandmother was a strong woman. She endured more than any of the women in our family could ever imagine. Yet she never let that weaken her faith in the least bit. In fact, when I would go into one of my crying fits or angry rages, she soothed me with just saying my name. She would always assure me that better times were ahead for me.

B. Blossom Lordman

Chapter 6

My Moses

I'll remind you that I was far from the perfect child . . . and I was promiscuous at a very young age. Yes, I did the old "sneaking around" with the neighborhood boys, because I thought it was the cool thing to do. Like many young girls, I thought it would make the boys like me.

I thought that my boyfriends would stay with me if I did, and let's be honest, I was just plain curious. I knew not to tell my grandparents that I was sexually active. It was like sex education just went straight out the window for me.

And in my curiosity, I got pregnant.

I was fourteen when Grandma took me to Dr.

McAnnally. I think that the man had been my pediatrician since I was born. Grandma had always taken me to the doctor every year before school started and this year was no different. I remember being so tired and wanting to sleep my summer away. Other than that, nothing seemed different to me.

The doctor did the usual check-up. He left the room, then came back in said, "Okay, young lady, we are looking good! Let's get you ready for the ninth grade!" My Grandmother then said, "Wait one minute, Doctor. I want you to give her a pregnancy test." The doctor and I looked at her like she was crazy! And of course, I immediately started to lie.

"Grandma, I'm not doing stuff like that!" I said. I begged and pleaded with her. But she wouldn't bend, and I could see irritation in the doctor's expression at the thought of me being pregnant.

I went to the bathroom with the little cup, all the while praying, "Oh, Dear God, please don't let me be pregnant. I promise never to have sex again!" I had promised this and promise that. Over and over I promised.

A few minutes later, the doctor came back into the room, slammed his clipboard down on the counter and growled, "Young lady, YOU ARE PREGNANT!"

It was like the world suddenly stopped! It felt as though someone was sucking the air out of the room, and I thought I would faint–either that or die! The look on my grandmother's face alone was enough to kill me.

I had disappointed her. *"Oh, no!"* I quickly thought. *"What is Granddaddy going to say?"* I didn't know how was I going to face him. I didn't know how I would face the church. I had no clue what I was going to do.

But the main question running through my mind at that moment was, *"Who in the heck is the father?"* I had no idea, and I was terrified.

I knew it had to be between two guys, but I was pretty sure it was the local neighborhood cutie. I just knew deep down in my soul that it was this guy because I actually loved him. He was really my friend, but we just happened to be too friendly. I prayed and prayed that the baby was his. After breaking the news, he and his family even began to accept the fact that the baby could be his.

Unfortunately, it wasn't him. It turned out to be the person I didn't want it to be—not because I didn't like him, but because of his age. And this time ya'll, I really had been a "fast girl."

The father of the baby lived across the street with a family member. I remember thinking he was cute, and on occasion I would flirt with him.

I remember the day that I got pregnant like it was yesterday.

On that day, I decided to walk over there, supposedly to see if a certain member of his family was home. She was not, but he invited me in anyway. I knew I should have turned around and gone back home, because if my grandparents had known I was over there alone with him, they would've killed me.

We talked for a few minutes, and for the life of me I can't remember how we got to *that* point. I can't even tell you how long it lasted, but I let it happen. We had sex, I promised him I wouldn't tell anyone, and that was it.

I never thought that I would get pregnant by *anyone*, let alone *him*. I ended up being the talk of the neighborhood. It was a mess. I was called a liar when it got around who the father might be. I'm pretty sure I was called some rather colorful names, but once again, no one looked at the fact that I was a child and he was a grown man.

I was also told that little girls have vivid imaginations, and that I *imagined* I had sex with him. This wasn't said by my grandparents, of course, but by nosey busybodies and sour old gossiping women.

I cried a lot during the beginning of my pregnancy. Not that I wasn't happy—well, as happy as a fourteen-year-old pregnant girl can be—but I just felt so alone. I couldn't go outside and play with the other little girls anymore. Many parents didn't want their daughters around me. Many women forbid their daughters from even being friends with me.

Was I a bad influence? Maybe. But was I ever looked at as a victim? I highly doubt it.

It didn't take long for it to sink in that I was actually pregnant! I was terrified, mainly of how my grandfather was handling the whole deal. Mama was furious. I expected her to be. There was talk of abortion. We even looked up the place in the phone book. Mama fussed, Grandma prayed, and I cried.

One day while looking through the phone book for a clinic, my grandfather came storming out of his room. With his big voice, he yelled, "Put those books up! Stop calling doctors! If she was woman enough to lie down to get it, she's gonna be woman enough to lie down and have it!" And that ended all talk of abortion.

I was actually happy that he stopped the abortion because I wanted my baby. I was both scared and excited. The fact that I was actually going to have a baby blew me away sometimes!

Sometimes I would rub my stomach and talk to my baby, and I slowly watched my teenage body transform to a womanly one.

Granddaddy eventually started talking to me again, which made the home life easier. I was so afraid to go to school that year, but imagine my surprise when I discovered that many others in my school were pregnant that year as well. I was not as alone as I thought.

School wasn't hard for me when I was pregnant, although there were a few teachers who thought I should have been enrolled in alternative school. I was never trouble to anyone; I was just pregnant. One teacher in particular said that my pregnancy took up attention in her class. Since I was not purposefully trying to be a distraction, her opinion didn't matter to me. I was there to get an education, and I would not let the opinions of others stop me.

I had some great friends in school, people that I still love like family to this day, and having people to lean on made my pregnancy seem to fly by. I enjoyed feeling my baby move inside me. Of course, there were still the whispers, stares, and accusations, but even at that tender age, I enjoyed my pregnancy.

One night as I was lying in bed, I felt my stomach start to tighten. I thought, *"No worries, maybe the little guy is stretching."* Then I started to feel pain and I got scared. I tiptoed downstairs to wake up Mama, who was staying there at the time. She came and lay in bed with me and rubbed my stomach.

By morning, the pains were worse. I heard Grandma tell Granddaddy that I was in labor. I have to say it was funny hearing my grandmother telling Mama, "Get her off of my couch before her water breaks!"

I was terrified! In my young mind, I thought I would just go into the hospital, push the baby out, and go back home. Oh, my goodness, I literally thought I was going to die! I was in labor for thirty-six hours! I just knew the Angel of Death was coming for me. No epidural, no painkillers– just a fourteen-year-old girl feeling like death!

After thirty minutes of pushing (and a nasty tear,) my little boy came into the world, weighing 6 pounds, 4 ½ ounces. Instantly, my life changed. Instantly, I fell in love. When I heard that little cry, all I wanted to do was hold him and never let him go! He was *the* most beautiful baby I had ever seen, and he was all mine. I named him after my grandfather. Despite the timing and the circumstances, God truly blessed me with my Moses.

After having my baby, my grandparents would not hear of me just quitting school and sitting around the house. At fifteen, I got my first job at Hardee's. My grandparents, my sister Sissy, and other ladies from my church would watch my son while I was at work and school.

At first, I didn't want to name him after my grandfather. (I thought maybe it was punishment for getting pregnant in the first place,) but I'm so happy that I did.

When my son turned three months old, I lost my grandfather to kidney failure. I was heartbroken because he wouldn't get to see his namesake grow up. He would be proud of my Moses; he turned out to be a great young man.

After having Moses, my main focus was to do two things in life: First, finish school, and second, give my son a family. I wanted the traditional family, with me, a husband, our kids, a house, two German Shepherds, and a happily ever after.

In my tenth or eleventh-grade year, I tried out for and made the Band Flag Team. I was so excited, and my grandmother didn't oppose it. I was happy to be in band. I thought this was a great opportunity for me because I still planned on going to college. Or so I thought.

Chapter 7

The Coach

I saw him on the sidelines of the football field. I was in the stands with my band members thinking, *"Who in the world is this big man on the field?"* I had seen him around the campus and in the hallways, but I didn't know who he was. However, I *did* know that I had to meet him! I started asking all of the football players just who this guy was.

Oh, all of the high school guys thought it was funny that I had a crush on this Teacher's Assistant/Coach, but I set out to meet him and I did just that. I remember giving a note to one of my classmates and begging him to give it to Coach.

It was a brave move on my part, because my classmate could have turned it into the principal instead and gotten me into trouble. But he didn't. My classmate came to me during lunch the next day and informed me that Coach wanted meet me in front of the school.

I was scared because I thought the man was going to get on my case for my actions, but he didn't. His words were, "I got your note and . . . I liked it."

We didn't immediately get into a relationship because, of course, we had to sneak around. I was so in love with everything about Coach–his walk, his talk, the way he dressed, and the way he smelled. I just knew that I had found my knight in shining armor.

He was amazing at first, buying me school clothes and gifts. He really bonded well with my little boy, and that was great because his biological father was nowhere to be found. My grandmother even felt like he was a good man for me.

Now my revised dream was to finish high school and

go to college while he coached the football team. I worked so hard to make it through school, and I was proud to be the only one of my mother's girls to get to high school. I was even prouder to be the only one to walk across the stage and accept my diploma.

Imagine the stone wall that I hit when I realized I was pregnant again. That's right, sixteen years old and pregnant with my second child.

Coach, my grandmother and I opted for an abortion immediately. That decision will haunt me for the rest of my life. I felt like I had no other choice, because I couldn't raise another child, and I certainly didn't want my beloved Coach to get into trouble.

Even now, I often sit and wonder what that sweet soul would have been like. I wonder if it was a boy or a girl. I beat myself up for a very long time after the abortion.

I have asked God for forgiveness over and over for aborting my baby, but to me, there had been no other way. It had just been my grandmother and I raising a little boy already. I had wanted the baby, but I couldn't add an extra burden like that on her.

Word started getting around about Coach and me. We'd both confided in people, a mistake we never should have made. Occasionally, various students would approach me and ask if something was going on between us; I would lie and say no. My grandmother sometimes let me go to his place and spend the night. I was so in love, and since I was rebelling and seeing him anyway at all hours of the night, she just gave up and let us be together.

⁓

As fate would have it, right in the middle of my eleventh-grade year I got pregnant. Again! This time, I refused to have an abortion. I couldn't do that to another baby. Like my grandfather had stated before, "I was woman enough to lie down and get with this baby, I was going to be woman enough to lie down and have it."

Coach was furious, but I just couldn't let this baby go. I figured he would just leave me alone to raise it like Moses's father had. And sometimes I wished he had, because he became very abusive.

The abuse started early with him. I think he felt trapped somehow. The first time he showed his anger, I didn't think anything of it. I blamed myself for making him mad.

We were going to go to the movies and my sister Karen was supposed to watch my little Moses. She wasn't home when we got to her house, so we didn't get to go.

For the life of me, I can't remember why he got angry, but boy did he get angry! He was driving so erratic, so crazy. I was afraid, so I was yelling at him to slow down. Once we pulled back into Grandma's driveway, I got out of the car. I should have walked in the house, but instead, I got back into the car to hit him. (Yes, the Gemini personality was showing out!) He grabbed me by my hair and we tussled. Then I ran in the house and he ran after me. I locked myself in the bathroom and he left, breaking my grandmother's screen door in the process.

That is the only time I will say it was my fault, because every other attack after that was not warranted.

Truthfully, abuse is never warranted.

Chapter 8

My Robbie

*T*hings began to smooth out between Coach and I, and he had no choice but to accept the pregnancy, so he started spending more time with me at my grandmother's.

I eventually moved out of Grandma's house when I was about seven to eight months pregnant with my Little Guy #2. I was eighteen and I didn't want to burden my grandmother with two babies.

Now mind you, Grandma lived in a very nice neighborhood called Kenilworth. I still drive by her old house whenever I visit Asheville. Nice tree-lined streets, beautiful houses. It was such a joy to wake up in that neighborhood because it was so quiet and serene. Well, I went from quiet and serene to an apartment in public housing.

This apartment complex was one of the popular drug spots. The day I moved in, I had never seen such ruckus in all my life! Don't get me wrong, I grew up in housing projects, and in my childhood, I had seen some real stuff! But this was the 90's and things had truly changed. On my first night alone, I heard gunshots and called Grandma in tears.

"Grandma, they're shooting!" I cried. "I hear gunshots!"

"Get on the floor!" she yelled into the phone. She came right over to pick me up, and she let me spend a few nights with her. But I knew I had to learn to be brave and live on my own.

Coach wasn't around much for the first part of my pregnancy. He spent some nights with me when I moved into my own apartment, but Moses and I spent most nights alone.

I was huge with my second child. I was pregnant with him all summer long and was completely miserable. I don't know how it is now, but public housing didn't have air conditioning back in the early 90's, so the place was hot beyond belief.

I kept myself busy by attending church and singing on the choir, trying to keep the connection with God.

I was massive by the time I hit my eighth month. My due date was September 3rd, but I tried everything in my power to go into labor early. I walked, I jumped rope, heck, I even drank castor oil, and got nothing! Not even a Braxton Hicks pain. I eventually gave up on the early labor trickery and decided to be patient.

Coach and I were asleep one night when all of a sudden I felt my water break. I called my sister to pick me up. We scrambled around, getting everything together. I called one of my friends to pick up Moses, and we high-tailed it to the hospital, only for them to send my back home.

They said it wasn't true labor. However, not even an hour later, I had to go back. After eighteen hours of labor (you bet your bottom dollar I had an epidural this time!) I had a C-Section because the little guy had taken his first poop inside. My Robbie weighed in at 8 pounds 1ounce.

He was the most precious baby–my little chub of joy! I adored him, just like I adored his father!

That night my happiness almost turned into tragedy. I was trying to breastfeed little Robbie. Once I got him latched on, I dozed off to sleep.

All of a sudden, it felt like somebody shook my hospital bed. Startled, I looked down at my baby, and my breast was covering his little nose and mouth. I was suffocating my baby! I quickly pulled my breast back. For a couple of seconds, he didn't take a breath. I shook him a little and just blew air in his face, and he took finally a deep breath. He was all right and breathing again. I thanked God over and over. It was truly a miracle that I awakened when I did.

My family was complete now. I had my two little boys, I had my Coach, and my little apartment. I was content.

Chapter 9

Tough Times

I decided to get my G.E.D. I was going to school and working in a deli at the same time. Coach didn't work. He stayed home and took care of the boys while I was working or at school. He took such good care of our children, so I didn't think anything of it, but some of my family members were furious that I was out working and maintaining my family when it should have been *him* who was working and me at home. I didn't care, just as long as I had my little family. That was all that mattered to me.

The real abuse began a little after Robbie was born. Coach would get so angry at me over little things, and sometimes over nothing. He would look for work but was unable to find anything. And I think that made him even angrier. Did he hit me a lot? No, but abuse is not always physical.

I remember one day in particular. For the life of me, I can't remember the reason for the argument, but things had gotten out of hand. I remember him grabbing me and pushing me up against the refrigerator. It was at that moment my grandmother came into my house. She was picking me up for choir practice.

She started yelling and shouting at him for pushing me. To my surprise, he started yelling and screaming at her too. He took his fist and broke my lamps. I mean he just shattered them. I remember pushing my grandmother out of the way so she wouldn't get hit by any of the debris.

With all the ruckus going on, I was trying to figure out just what I did to piss him off. He then snatched up my baby and walked out the door. This would not be the last time he had held my son from me as punishment. He brought him back and apologized, and I forgave. Sadly, this would become a pattern for us for about seven years.

I endured a lot of mental abuse from Coach. But I loved him, and all I wanted was for my boys to be raised in a traditional family. Not only was he mentally and physically abusive, but he was also a cheater.

It seemed as though he went for anyone that I befriended. Oh, I'm positive there were more, but two women in particular come to mind.

Girl # 1. I met her at the WIC office when I was still pregnant with Robbie. We immediately hit it off because we both were huge! After we'd had our babies, we started making our WIC appointments at the same time.

She wasn't from Asheville, so I showed her which stores to go to use her WIC vouchers. A good friend indeed, right?

Wrong!

Little did I know that behind my back, Coach had slept with her. He started driving her car and dropping her off at work. I mean, it was all just right in my face. This was the first time (that I know of) that he'd slept around on me, so I forgave him and took him back.

Girl # 2. I was preparing for Robbie's birthday party. I believe it was his second birthday. A few days (or weeks) before, I met this young lady–we will call her Jane. She seemed nice, and she was new to the area. I've always been a sucker for meeting new people, so I decided to befriend her. Little did I know that she would become a thorn in my side, and remain there for a *very* long time.

I invited her to help me set up for Robbie's' party. We talked and didn't seem to have much in common, but she was friendly. I introduced her to Coach. And thus, the regular cheating saga *and* my addiction to food began.

I would be upstairs in bed sometimes and hear Coach talking to someone. Then I'd go downstairs to find her in my house, talking to him like she lived there. I was timid and didn't say much, so she started getting braver, pulling up in front of my apartment to pick him up. And he would just go!

It became very embarrassing because all the neighbors began to talk. Soon they began to laugh. At that point, I decided to start seeing other people as well. I felt that if he could do it, then so could I. When he would go out the front door, I would take my kids and sneak out the back. I know it wasn't the right thing to do, but if he was giving another female his attention, then I would have to seek attention in other places as well. But I found no real happiness from the situation.

Once when I said something to Coach about going out with Jane all of the time and leaving me and the kids home, he blew up at me, so I stopped saying anything about it because I was afraid of him.

I soon developed my own way to cope.

Whenever he left, I would eat. Cookies, Little Debbie cakes, candy, or anything else sweet. I would eat until I was completely stuffed, and then fall asleep. Food became my comforter.

In the projects, there was a "Candy Truck/Bus" that sold everything from single cigarettes to fried chicken. It was an old, school bus, transformed into a store. I would walk up to wherever it was parked and buy a bag of junk food and a pack of cigarettes (I can't remember if it was Newport or Marlboro Lights.) I would then return home and eat all the junk food I purchased, smoke me a square, and then drift off to sleep in my own little world.

$\sim$

Things got pretty bad between Coach and I–bad and weird, really. I could go on and on about everything that man had done to me.

We ended up losing the apartment, and I moved back into my grandmother's house. He stayed with his folks for a while but ended up getting an apartment in another complex.

To me, this is really where he and Jane began to be evil in my sight, because he would do sick things to me, and she seemed to aid him.

While the boys and I were living with Grandma, Coach and I would always go back and forth, arguing about something, anything! He didn't help when it came to child support, so Grandma watched the boys while I worked.

One evening I asked Grandma to watch the boys while I went out with some friends. Now mind you, we didn't have cell phones back then. When I got home, I saw that my grandmother had been crying and I thought something was wrong with one of the boys.

She told me that Coach came by the house looking for me. When he learned that I wasn't there, he pushed past her, grabbed Robbie (he would never take Moses, as Moses was not his biological Son), and got into the car where Jane was waiting, and they drove off. The next day I had to beg and plead for them to return my son to me. Under *his* conditions, *she* brought Robbie back.

I tried so hard to go on with my life, but he just wouldn't let me. Every time I would move, he'd find me, showing up unannounced, and bullying me as always.

⌒

You would think with all of the sleeping around and cheating and abuse, I would have left Coach completely. No, I married him instead. Yes, I did, because I thought I could save my relationship and keep my family together.

But despite all my efforts, Jane would still be a thorn

in my side.

The week after we got married at the court house, I moved into Coach's apartment, and I was instantly sorry. He lost what little respect he'd had left for me the minute I married him. Jane's mother lived in the same complex, so I would see them riding out together all of the time. He'd just do it right in my face. But I knew not to say anything because whenever I did decide to stand up for myself, he'd beat me up, right in front of Jane and her mother.

Like I said before, I could sit here and name every single thing Coach and Jane did to me. But that is another book in itself. It stung seeing them together all of the time; after all, he was *my* husband. But Jane just dug in her heels and would not let go.

So, I finally did. I found the courage to leave him for good.

It was tough for me, because I was by myself now, moving from place to place, constantly having to fight Coach over my kids (it almost seemed as if Jane wanted them for her own.) He never worked, so there was still no child support money.

As time went on, I got used to Coach and Jane being together. I was over it and just wanted to go on with my life. I was still having trouble finding my own apartment, so I stayed with family members. Let me say this: I've found that family members will treat you like crap when you're down on your luck, and it's better to stay in a shelter.

To compensate and soothe the emotional hurt, I started eating too much. I would buy boxes of snack cakes and wait until everybody in the house was asleep. When the coast was clear, I would sit and eat and eat. Sometimes I fell asleep with food in my mouth, and would wake up with crumbs in my bed. Food was my companion!

B. Blossom Lordman

Chapter 10

The Marriage That Should Never

Have Happened

*F*or a while, I had to let the boys go and stay with Coach and Jane because I couldn't find a stable place to live. I moved in with my cousin. We both worked in manufacturing. She didn't charge me too much to stay there and we got along great.

That is until she introduced me to husband number two. We will call him Ben.

Ben was all chocolate and smart, with a beautiful smile and a good talk. I fell for him instantly. He was such a gentleman–and just the type of quirky guy I needed. Little did I know that he would bring me seven years of hell!

I didn't know he was a full-on addict! He never let on. He never let one hint slip that he was addicted to crack cocaine. I tried so hard to help him kick the habit, because again, I wanted a family for my boys. Instead, I gave them seven years of the worst rollercoaster ride of their little lives, and I will forever have to live with that.

When things were good, they were really good. But when things were bad, it was pure hell! There were times when Ben would be missing for days. He would take all of our bill money and just smoke it up. The power would be turned off, and eviction notices started coming. The stress of it all caused me to have two miscarriages. But then the good Lord knew what I was going through, and I would *not* have been able to care for another child at that time.

Nothing was safe in the house either. I would come home from work to find that Ben had pawned our TVs and the kids video games. It all grew to be too much! There were times when he would take the car for days, leaving me with no way to work, and no way to get groceries for the kids, basically leaving me stuck.

As Ben's addiction to crack spiraled out of control, so did my food addiction. He started getting into trouble with the law, robbing convenience stores, stealing from work. You name it he did it. Through all of his incarcerations, food was my companion. I was so depressed.

I stuck by him for seven years before finally deciding to give up on the marriage. I decided to let the streets have him. I didn't need that kind of husband.

Instead, food became my husband.

I started to binge. Though I never purged, I would just go into a binging frenzy. I would go to the store and purchase all of my favorite snacks. I would get the kids what they wanted, but I never let them see just how much I had gotten for myself. Then I would wait until nighttime, go into my room, and eat every single piece of candy, every bag of Doritos, every package of Little Debbie cakes, and then wash it all down with grape soda. I would follow it up by smoking one or two cigarettes, and drift off into the arms of my love;

food!

Eating was like having sex for me. Binging was *the* best feeling in the world at that time, because I had no one.

After the breakup of my second marriage, I lived alone for a little while, falling deeper into binging. There was no one to hide my addiction from then. I was alone. I could eat as much as I wanted, as often as I wanted. Food had become my *Main Squeeze*! Oh, I had short-lived relationships here and there. Some ended badly, and some partings were clean and we still remain friends today.

I was so unhappy with my weight. I would always start a weight loss plan and quickly fall off. I would see commercials for weight loss clinics, and then go check them out only to have them ask me the dreaded question, "How much can you afford to pay?"

There were times when I would cry myself to sleep because I knew I needed to do something about getting the weight off. Eventually, I just gave up and pushed it to the back of my mind.

I was content being single. I had everything I needed–

a job, a little apartment, car, and *food*! By this time, I was working at a local debt collection firm, and I wasn't really looking to date anyone.

B. Blossom Lordman

Chapter 11

Blinded by Stupidity

I happened to meet a guy. We'll call him Mick. I should have known from the jump not to get involved with him because he just looked like trouble. But I was lonely. I needed the company of a man, and that's all I wanted in the beginning–company.

Mick wasn't really anything to call home to Mama about, but he was very street, and very interesting to me. His walk, his accent, everything about him was interesting! I was never the "street" type of woman, because I was raised in the church.

Immediately, his drug use surfaced. I seemed to attract these types for some reason. I tended to look past the bad in people and tried to bring out the good. My grandmother always told me, "Blossom, you can't save everybody, that's Jesus's job." Would I listen?

Of course not! In fact, I tried to save him so much that I followed him out of town. My boys were living with their father and stepmother in Asheville, so there was nothing holding me back.

When we got to New Jersey, Mick was supposed to help me find a job and a place and then we'd part ways. I was helping him get back home, so he was *supposed* to help me start a new life for myself. I didn't want a life with *him*, I just wanted to try living in a new state for a while and meet some new people.

When we got to our destination, reality slapped me in the face. Literally! He had me hanging around drug dealers and guns. I was sleeping on folk's couches, living in houses with no running water. We only had a little money, so we were forced to eat in soup kitchens. He would leave me with his friends, and then go to other women's houses to eat. There were times when I would eat his leftovers because we were down to nothing.

It was ironic that I was the one who ended up helping him to get a job. We applied for the same job at a collection agency where he was previously employed. They hired me and not him, so I had to beg to get him a position once I got my foot in the door.

Yes, I was once again trying to play the savior. It was a rough time and I knew absolutely no one but Mick. Did he appreciate the help I'd given him? No. He showed his appreciation by putting me out of the house with nowhere to go.

Now I was born and raised in Asheville, North Carolina and had moved to Greenville, South Carolina before making that move up north. I knew nothing, absolutely nothing about New Jersey.

Well, one night, we decided to get a room. We were supposed to just be getting food and drinks (we finally had some money,) and then go back to the room. Mick's friend called and told him that he had a girl he wanted him to meet. And that very instant, he dropped me!

He told me that I would have to find somewhere else to stay for the night, because he wanted to "chill" with this little honey. I couldn't believe it! I just couldn't believe that he would leave me high and dry just for sex with someone else!

I drove around on this rainy night, praying to find somewhere to stay. I found an expensive Holiday Inn to stay for the night. I was feeling so down, I called friends and family, crying about my situation. They begged me to come back home, but I didn't want to. I wanted to show them all that I could handle it on my own.

I decided to stay, and I soon found some people to help me. How many of you know that God always has a ram in the bush? I had been desperately looking for a place to stay. I already had a job, and all I needed was a place to sleep, just until I could get my own apartment. That's when I met this sweet girl. We'll call her Blondie.

Blondie allowed me to stay in her spare bedroom. We worked in Thorofare, New Jersey at the time, but she lived close by in Penns Grove.

Blondie was bold, beautiful, and loud, and her house was a regular party spot. The first night at her house was a culture shock for me. Thinking about it, I have to smile, because she was everything I wanted to be. She had a boyfriend at the time named Pip, and he was a true character! There was never a dull moment in her house. But I knew I couldn't stay there for long because I was never the partying type. Did I join in? Yes, I did! She showed me a good time, taking me to clubs, drinking, laughing dancing. But this just wasn't the life that I had planned for myself.

I stayed with Blondie for a couple of weeks, trying to save my money to either get my own place, or get out of New Jersey. I was on the fence about going back to South Carolina, but fate would make my decision for me.

One cool night, Mick called and asked me to come and chill with him. He was living with a friend over in Wilmington, Delaware. I knew that I should have kept myself in New Jersey, but honestly, I needed the attention of a man that night. I was lonely, and he was the only one I knew.

I got all dressed and headed back over to Delaware. He invited me upstairs to hang out. We talked and laughed for a while, and then we decided to go pick up some Vodka. Once we got back to the apartment, more of his friends had shown up. I didn't think anything of it, because he invited me over to hang out with *him*.

After a few drinks, Mick told me that one of his friends wanted to "get with me." I objected at first, but the more I drank, the more he pressed, and I finally gave in and said yes. He left the room and went downstairs and sent his friend in.

The room was dark, so I really couldn't see who entered the room; all I saw was a silhouette. When the friend came in and we started, I noticed that the door opened a second time, then a third, then a fourth. I was completely drunk and confused as to what was going on. When I felt more than one pair of hands on me, I knew what was going on.

I didn't know what to think, what to do. So many questions ran through my head. What do I say? Do I try to run? Do I ask them to stop? Do I scream? What do I do? One of the guys started to get rough with me and I asked where Mick was. One of the friends said that he was downstairs. I got up, trying to cover my extra-large body with my hands and went downstairs where Mick was on the couch, stoned out of his mind.

I said to him, "Mick, please come up there, please. I'm scared! I don't want to go back up there!" He took my hand, led me back upstairs, and scolded them for scaring me. I still couldn't see because it was dark in the house. I heard one of the guys say, "You better tell her how we do it up here, Mick." What's sad is Mick turned around a left me in the room with them. He just walked out and left me. I begged them not to be so rough, and I told them I would cooperate. I just wanted it all to end. I wanted it over with.

I don't know if one of them suddenly got a guilty conscience, or if he felt sorry for me, but he stopped. He told the rest, "That's enough; get off of her." On his command, they stopped.

Oh, hindsight is a clever teacher, because now it is all clear to me. I had just paid Mick's drug debt.

I cleaned myself up, and got out of there. Once I was outside, I ran. I had no idea where I was going, but I knew for sure that I was not going to the cops. I was getting the hell out of Delaware!

I was frantic, not knowing which way to go. Then I remembered; Blondie's ex-boyfriend told me where he lived, and it happened to be right around the corner. I jumped into my Ford Escort and peeled out of there.

I ran to the ex-boyfriend's door, and thankfully, they let me in. I was a mess—crying uncontrollably, afraid and humiliated. I just wanted to get back to South Carolina as soon as possible. The ex-boyfriend ran outside and called for Big Johnny. All I kept hearing was, "Hey, go get Big Johnny. Somebody go get Big Johnny!"

In my head, all I could think was, *"Who in the heck is Big Johnny, and why is he being summoned?"* I didn't know what to think. Was I going to have to fight? Was Big Johnny coming to harm me or protect me? After all I had just been through, I was desperately praying for protection.

Big Johnny came through the door, instructing everyone to get me up off the floor. He asked me what happened, and through my tears, I told him. He and

Blondie's ex were livid! They immediately set out to defend my honor, to "take care" of the thugs that had treated me so badly.

I begged them not to go up there, because I knew what type of thugs these guys were, and I sure didn't want anyone to get hurt. I only had one request. I needed help to get back to South Carolina. At that point, I didn't care what I had to do. I even offered to leave them my old broken-down car if they would only purchase me a Greyhound bus ticket.

Big Johnny promised he would get me home. He fed me, and then offered me his bed, never trying to touch me, or harm me in any way. He truly protected me.

The next morning, we all agreed that I would leave my car in Delaware, and they would buy me a Greyhound ticket back to Greenville. Not only did I have to leave my car, but I left all of my pictures, jewelry, and my grandmother's jewelry box. But at that moment, I didn't care what I had to leave, as long as I got back to South Carolina.

It was soon time for me to board the bus. Johnny seemed sad that I was leaving. He kept telling me how worried he was about me. We exchanged numbers and hugged. I promised him that I would stay in touch when I got back home. He promised that he would come down and visit me.

As the Bus pulled off, I broke down in tears. I was mad, sad, and afraid. Any emotion that I could feel, I felt. I was sad because I really didn't want to go back to South Carolina. I honestly wanted to make a life for myself in New Jersey or Delaware. I was mad because I let myself get tricked by Mick, and let myself get hurt by his thug friends. I should have been smarter than I had been. I should have been wiser. And I was afraid because I was going back home with nothing, and I felt totally humiliated.

Chapter 12

Knight in Shining Armor

I arrived back in South Carolina on a Saturday afternoon. I felt that this had to be the lowest point in my life. I had to go and live with Karen, her husband and kids, and Mama. Needless to say, I was miserable.

Life in my sister's household was sometimes unbearable. She had strict house rules and kept close watch over the food, which was not a good situation for a food addict. I would find myself sometimes sneaking food, but never sneaking so much that she would notice. I was an extra mouth in her household at the time because I came with nothing. My sister and I would get into arguments sometimes, and to get out of the house and reduce stress, I would go and spend time at the local neighborhood hangouts.

I began to drink and party with my newfound friends/family. They were a breath of fresh air and I relished being away from my sister's house. Beer became my favorite drink. It was nothing for me to sit and drink almost a full six-pack.

Big Johnny kept his word about checking up on me. He had called the first night I got home, and I had been happy to hear from him. He began calling me every day, sometimes several times a day. He offered to send me money because I didn't have a job, and things were getting kind of sticky at Karen's.

Johnny and I became very close friends. He eventually asked if he could come down and visit. Of course, my answer was yes. We made plans for him to come in the spring.

Johnny's bus arrived on a Sunday afternoon and I was very happy to see him. I took him to meet my family, and they were skeptical, but I wasn't. I knew in my heart that Johnny was a good person. He offered to pay for a room at a local hotel for a week, and I jumped at the chance to finally get out of my sister's house for a while.

Johnny and I found we had so much in common that it was easy to relax with each other. For the first time in my life, I was being treated the way a woman should be treated. Johnny spoiled me. Anything that I asked for, he would get for me.

We found that we loved the same music, sometimes sitting in front of the radio for hours playing music and singing along. I enjoyed our time together. He fed into my addictions and added another in the mix: marijuana. It went well with my food addiction!

Johnny seemed to like to feed me. Yes, *feed* me, because he knew food made me happy. Sometimes we would sit and order large amounts of food. We were never able to eat it all, but we sure tried. We both seemed to find happiness in food, and each other.

Johnny was only supposed to stay with me for two weeks and then go back to Delaware, but we fell for each other hard, and I didn't want him to go. When the time came for him to leave, he asked if he could just go ahead and stay with me in South Carolina. My answer was a definite yes!

We only had to stay with my sister for one week. Then we got an efficiency apartment and began our life together.

Chapter 13

The Life of Blossom and Johnny

either Johnny nor I worked. Johnny was receiving unemployment benefits from his previous job in New Jersey, and it was enough to sustain us for a while. We stayed in our efficiency for about four months, and we got along well. There were hardly any disagreements between us, and if there were, it was because I was acting spoiled.

We eventually decided we needed more space and wanted to move into an apartment complex across the street from where we were staying. Now mind you, neither of us had an active job, so we didn't know how we were going to obtain the apartment.

The landlord was an angel. She worked with us and let us have the place. It had been so long since I'd had a real place of my own, and Johnny and I were so excited to move in! We didn't have any furniture and we didn't care! All we had was an air mattress and each other, and that's all we needed.

After we got settled, our apartment became the hangout spot for a while. I would cook big Sunday dinners and invite family and friends over. We would have cookouts by the pool, and we enjoyed doing so. Life with Johnny was simply awesome. My boys even fell in love with him, mainly because they were happy to finally see their mama happy.

Johnny helped me get through some real rough spots. He would sit and listen when I told him about my past. Not only would he listen, but he would allow me to go through my fits of rage, comforting me and reassuring me that everything was okay, and promising me he would never let anything happen to me again.

So much happened in the first year of our relationship. My oldest son was deployed twice, to Afghanistan and Iraq, and I had never been so scared in of my life! I still thank God daily for protecting my son, and for sending him back to me. Even though your children grow up, you never stop worrying about them, especially when they are so far away.

Thank you, Moses, for your service.

B. Blossom Lordman

Chapter 14

My Miracle

I was at the point in my life where I could finally relax a little. I didn't have to work, and my boys were grown and out on their own. Moses was no longer deployed and was now living in California. Robbie was living in Asheville with his father and stepmother, sometimes coming to spend a few weeks with me. Johnny and I still had friends and family over from time to time, and things were beginning to finally balance out. Well, everything except my weight.

I was happy therefore I ate! I'm pretty sure I was at my heaviest at that time. I didn't have a scale and didn't care to own one, I just knew I was very heavy, and I didn't let it bother me. I was finally having some peace, some normalcy.

We eventually invited Johnny's mother to visit from New Jersey, and at that time my stepsister Katrina and her boys were staying with us. (I have a lot of stepsiblings) We had a house full, but since it was just Johnny and I, it was fine.

While Johnny's mother was visiting, I became ill. I didn't know what was wrong, all I knew was I couldn't keep any food down; food didn't even taste good to me, which was rare, because we all know how much I loved food. I got so sick that I decided to go to the hospital. At this time, the H1N1 Swine Flu was spreading across the country like wildfire and I was certain I had it!

Johnny and I rushed to the hospital. When we got there, I explained all my symptoms to the nurse. They had me do the old "pee in a cup," and they brought in a dye for me to drink so they could do a scan of my stomach. I couldn't even keep it down.

Just as the nurse was bringing in more dye to drink, The ER doctor rushed in and stopped me from drinking it. I remember so vividly the grin on his face. I was getting kind of peeved, because I felt like I was dying and this doctor was smiling at me.

"What is it?" I asked. "What's wrong with me? Do I have the Swine Flu?"

He didn't say anything, he just shook his head no, and then looked down at my stomach. I was confused for a split second, and then it hit me.

"I'm pregnant?" I exclaimed.

He nodded. "Yes!"

I didn't know what to say, I didn't know what to think, and for a second, I thought that I would faint. I looked over at Johnny and he had this blank look on his face. I'm laughing as I write this because it was so surreal. I said to Johnny, "Oops!" You have to realize Johnny had grown children as well.

He said to the doctor, "Well, you just ruined my whole damned day, Doc!"

The doctor began to apologize, asking if it was a *bad* thing that I was pregnant.

I quickly told him that this was a welcomed pregnancy. The surprise is that God waited eighteen long years to make this miracle happen. My children were grown–ages eighteen and twenty-one! I couldn't believe I was going to be a new mommy again!

I quickly grabbed the phone and called Mama and my sisters. No one could believe it, except for two people: my stepsister Katrina and Johnny's mother. Somehow, they knew!

Chapter 15

My Johnathyn

My pregnancy was not an easy one, and my doctors classified me as "high risk" because of my age, weight, and blood pressure problems. Eventually, I developed preeclampsia and was put on bed rest. I had several ultra sounds to make sure the baby was okay, so I knew I was having a boy. Johnny and my friends were awesome. My friends gave me my very first baby shower and my sister Karen even stepped up to help.

I had to deliver my baby boy early because my blood pressure wouldn't stay down, and I was on constant bed rest. The doctors were afraid of toxemia. I remember being so scared because it had been so long since I had given birth, and I was terrified. Johnny was afraid to stay with me during the labor, so I called my sister to be with me.

On June 29th, 2010 by way of C-Section, and weighing in at 5lbs 7oz, my sweet little miracle made his entrance into this world, and he changed my life forever.

When they finally delivered little Johnathyn, I held my breath until he took his first. I didn't have to hold it for long because I heard him breathe; I heard him cry. They brought him over to me, and when I looked at that sweet face, I was in love.

Now my life was complete. I didn't need anything else. I had my Johnny, and my oldest boys were safe and sound where they were. I had my own place, and now I had my new baby boy. This little angel changed my life in more ways than one.

Chapter 16

Normalcy

*I*t had been so long since I was truly happy. In fact, I don't think I had ever been that happy– so happy in fact, my weight began to rise. If I was not at my heaviest at this point, I was sure close to it. Johnny and I were adapting to being new parents again, and along with the happiness came the extra weight.

All was well, except one thing. Neither one of us was employed. His unemployment benefits were beginning to run out. We both looked for work, and I found employment first. I was lucky enough to find a full-time job right across the street at a drug store.

I hadn't worked in a very long time, and I was

apprehensive about leaving my son every day. I worked mostly day shifts. Johnny eventually found a job at the local chicken plant, so everything was beginning to balance out.

I loved spending time with my little baby while his dad was at work. During that time, it was just little Johnathyn and me. While I cooked and cleaned, he played happily. Everything was definitely working out!

Chapter 17

My Weight Becomes a Problem

When I say that my weight became a problem, I mean a health problem, a dangerous health problem. I had stopped smoking cigarettes when I got pregnant with Johnathyn, but quickly picked it back up after he was born. My weight was never that important to me, but I began to have health issues.

I was always running to the hospital because of blood pressure spikes. When I would get to the hospital, my numbers would be 200/116, sometimes higher! I had always had problems with my blood pressure, but it was worsening.

I remember going to the ER and having the nurse tell

me that I needed to lose weight. It didn't hit me like a ton of bricks or anything because I already knew that. She gave me some advice on how to eat better and cook better. Like always, after getting my medication and leaving the hospital, I went back to eating bad, smoking cigarettes, and just not caring.

At my doctor's appointments, they always fussed about my A1C levels being too high. Yes, they said the same stuff over and over. "Lose weight, stop smoking, blah, blah, blah."

I never really thought about my weight being a problem, because it never stopped me from working and doing my job. I was strong, I could lift heavy boxes, I *felt* healthy, and that was all that mattered.

One night Johnny and I were talking and he said to me, "You know, you stop breathing sometimes when you're asleep."

That startled me, because sometimes I would wake up gasping for air and not knowing why. I told my doctor about it, and we scheduled an appointment for a sleep test. My health was spiraling out of control.

My health and weight didn't stop me from being a

good mom though. However, it did start to concern me. I was a teen when I had my older children, but I was heading into my 40's with my youngest son.

B. Blossom Lordman

Chapter 18

The Final Straw

*J*ohnathyn had become mobile. It was not a problem when he started crawling; the problem came when he started walking. He would get into everything and pick up anything that wasn't nailed down. Anything that he picked up would also quickly go into his mouth.

One day after work I decided to make dinner. I was tired, my feet were hurting, but I had to get dinner on the table. I sat down at the kitchen table to peel potatoes while Johnathyn played happily on the floor.

While dinner was cooking, I went into the living room and sat on the couch to give my feet a rest. I noticed that Johnathyn was walking toward the kitchen table, arms stretched out like he was reaching for something. I looked up and the knife was on the edge of the table.

I called out him, "Johnathyn, don't touch!" He didn't listen, of course. I went to get up off of the couch to get him, and I couldn't get up. No, I wasn't sick or hurt, but I was just too heavy to even get up off the couch.

He got closer to the knife, and I kept trying to get off that couch. I rocked once, then twice, holding onto the arm of the couch for leverage. Still, I couldn't get up. All I could see in my mind was my baby getting a hold of that knife.

I eventually gave up and rolled onto the floor, and I crawled over to the table and grabbed my toddler before he could grab the knife. I sat there for a minute and just looked at my baby, thanking God for letting me get there in time.

That was the day that I decided it was time for me to do something about my weight. I had a little talk with myself. *"I have to be here to raise my son. I have to be here to finish what God started. He trusted me with this little gift, and I have to be here!"*

Besides Johnny, I didn't trust–and still don't trust–anybody to raise Johnathyn. If anything happened to me, what would happen to him? What kind of man would he turn out to be without his mommy? How would his father raise him without me?

Oh, yes! The time had come for me to change.

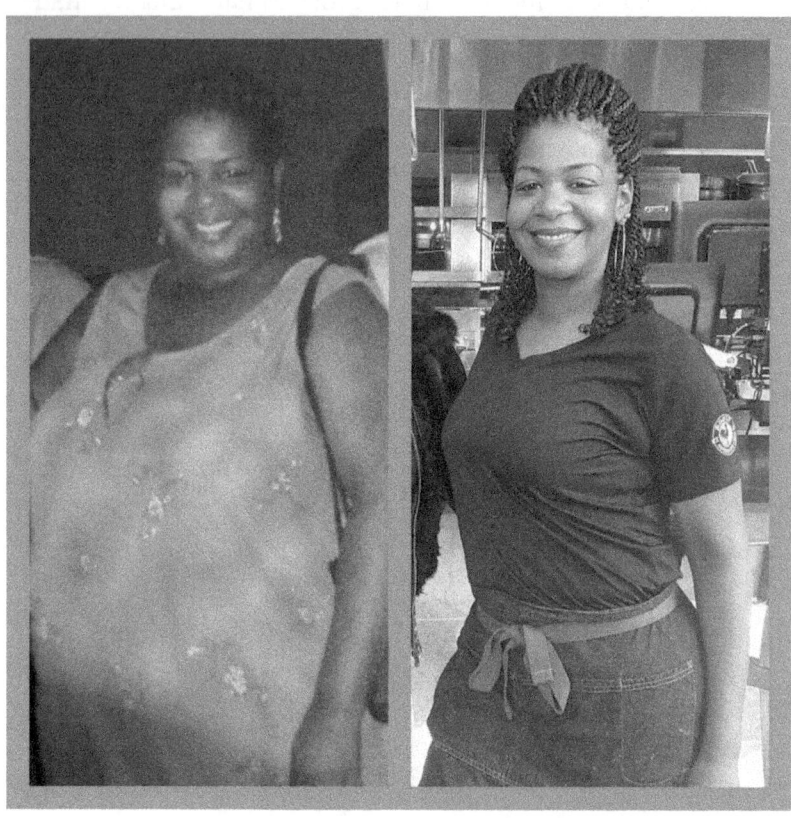

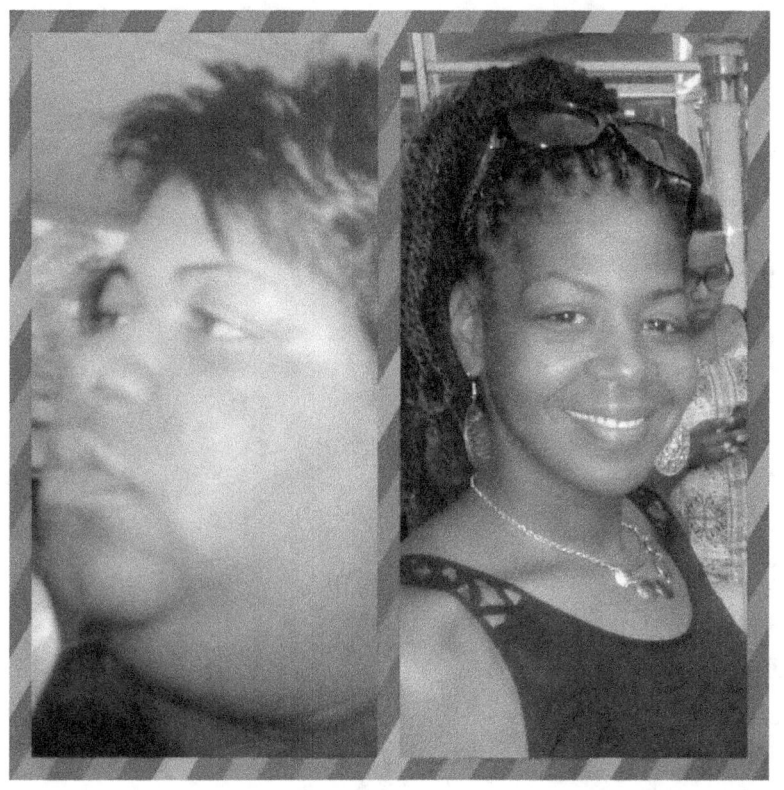

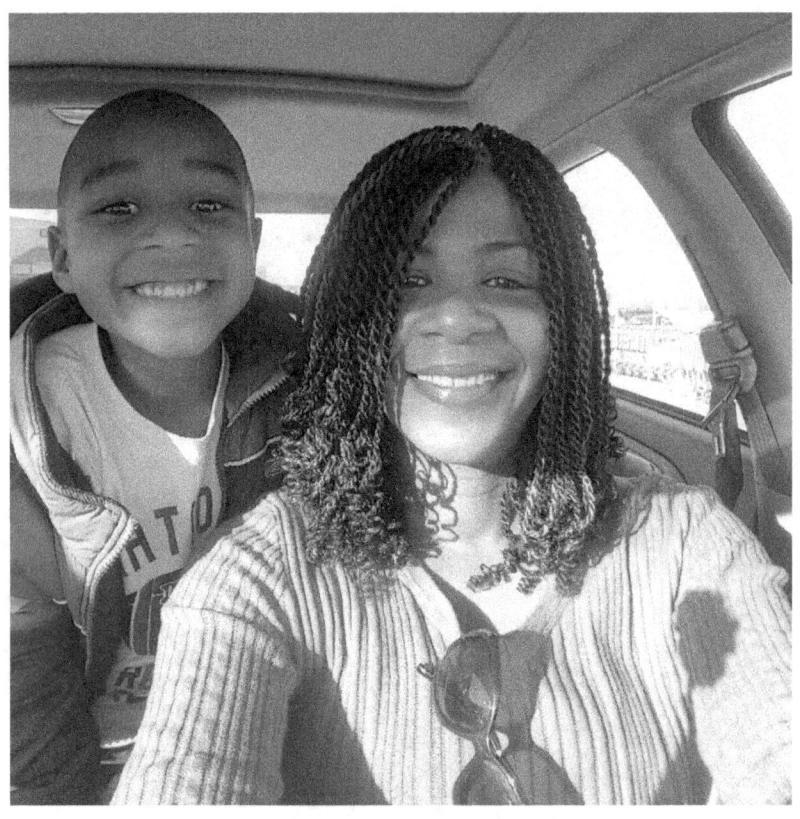

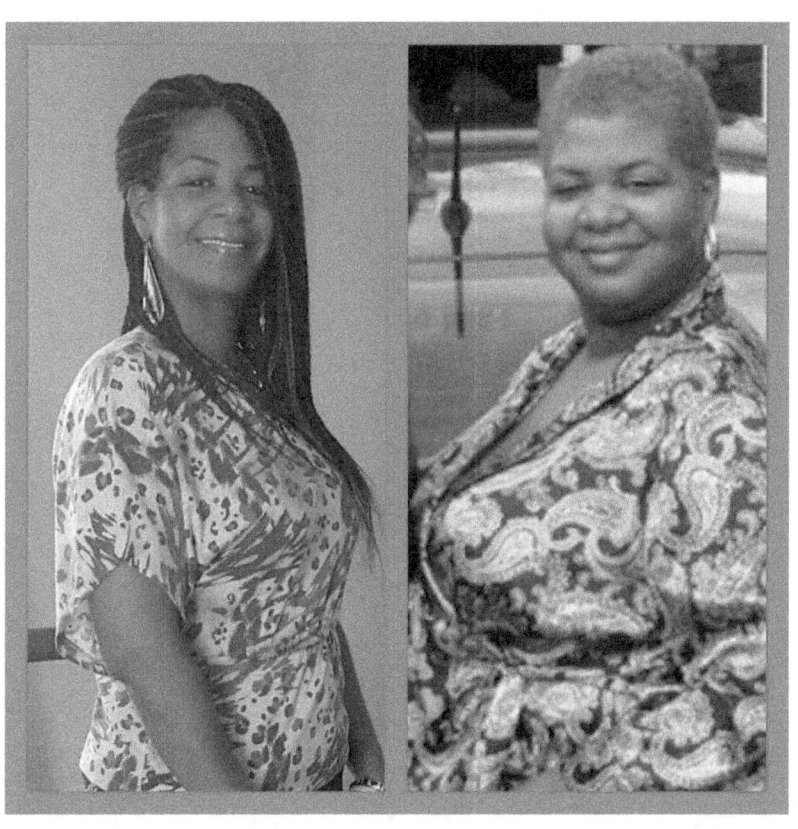

B. Blossom Lordman

Chapter 19

Where Do I Start?

M y change was not immediate. I didn't suddenly start eating super healthy, and truthfully, I didn't change anything. I was a cashier at a drug store, so in my down time, I would read health magazines, trying to figure out a way to get myself healthy.

I had tried dieting in the past, but I always failed. In fact, I had lost as much as fifty pounds, but I gained it all back. This time had to be different. This time I had to get this weight off and keep it off. The more I read, the more I learned.

My diet at the time consisted of fried chicken, pork chops, potatoes, burgers, hotdogs . . . I could go on and on. I would have a Filet O' Fish meal for lunch, and then back it up with a box of chocolates.

It was so easy to stand at the cash register and eat candy and chips in my down time, and I had a lot of down time, because we were not a busy store. I think that may have been the hardest foe to fight in the beginning of my lifestyle change. Being around all of that junk food was like putting a heroin addict in a room full of heroin. I knew something had to change, but I just didn't know where to begin.

Chapter 20

A Trip to the Gym

(Thank you, Katrina!)

I hadn't thought about any form of fitness. I had taken on a more strenuous position at the grocery store, but that was about it. I was mobile and I worked every day, but I had no idea where to start with exercise. Then one day my little sister Katrina asked me to go to the gym with her.

I had tried working out in the past, but I always gave up. Since she didn't want to go alone, I decided to go with her. She took me to a spinning class. I had never heard of a spin class, but I went along with it.

When I walked into the gym, surprisingly, I did not

feel intimidated. I was in awe at all of the bright lights and loud music. I saw people running on treadmills and lifting weights. There was a buzz about the place that just felt interesting.

We walked into the spin room and it was amazing to me. All of the bicycles were lined in a row with mirrors everywhere, and the music was very loud and upbeat. Everyone seemed so nice and inviting.

The time came for the class to begin, and as soon as I started to pedal, I wanted to kill Katrina. It was the hardest thing I had ever done in my life! I was still a two pack a day smoker, so I felt as though my lungs were going to pop.

My weave was sweating out, my heart was about to beat out of my chest, and I kept throwing my sister evil looks. Every time I would give her the death look, she would smile at me. No, her smile was not to laugh at me, but to encourage me.

Her smile said to me, "You can do this, just keep it up." My legs burned and my heart raced, but one thing was for sure. I did not get off of that bike. I made it through the entire class. It was then that I fell in love with working out.

After that spin class, I was hooked. I wanted to do more. I wanted to go again. I was ready to begin my lifestyle change. I began to really dig in and research how to lose weight. I didn't want to diet. I wanted to change.

I think I subscribed to every health magazine known to man and I would read every page. If the article seemed interesting, or if I questioned the article, I would Google. Google became a wonderful tool for me. It was beneficial in my lifestyle change.

I would Google everything from "What is obesity doing to my body?" to "What are the health benefits of exercise?" I went to the library and did researches on weight loss. I had to find out all I could; I had to get this right. If I intended to be here for my sons and grandchildren, I had to lose this weight.

With all of my reading and research, I came up with a plan for myself. Thank God my plan worked. It was all trial and error, but the plan God set for me changed my lifestyle forever.

Let me tell you how I lost 110 pounds. Let me tell you

how I beat food addiction. And let me tell you how I turned HURT into HEALTH!

Chapter 21

Portion Control

Why is it important to control portion sizes?

Portion control is understanding how much a **serving size** of food is and how many calories or how much food energy a **serving** contains. **Portion control** is **important** for body weight management as the weight is defined by the total calorie intake. **(Wikipedia)**

The first thing I learned, of course, was portion control. I didn't immediately change *what* I ate, but I changed *how much* I ate. I purchased measuring cups, spoons, and bowls. I had to learn what a true portion was.

In America, we tend to eat out of bigger plates, and we fill them up, not measuring what a true portion is. When I began to use measuring tools, I found that I was indeed filling my plate with too much food. Eventually, I started eating out of smaller plates and bowls.

I learned to read nutrition labels. If the label called for ¼ cup for my portion, then that's what I ate. If the label said 2 pieces of bread was a portion, again, that's what I would eat, and no more. I also learned to use my hand as a guide for measuring out my food.

When I prepared my plate, I made sure to fill half of my plate with veggies, leaving a little room for starches and meat.

When I went out to eat, I would immediately ask for a to-go box to put half of my food in. Restaurants tend to serve huge plates that are full of fat and calories. So, I would try to limit how many times a week I intended to eat out.

Was I hungry at first? Yes, because I was so used to eating until I got stuffed. My stomach had to get used to the correct portions of food. So, when I got hungry, the first thing I did was to drink a big glass of water, just to make sure that I wasn't thirsty.

When I get hungry in between meals, I eat healthier snacks. I used to eat so much junk food, and it was nothing for me to grab a bag of Doritos, candy, and a soda, especially at work. I made a conscience effort to eat better.

Instead of those chips, I grab an apple or almonds, or peanuts. Instead of a sugary soda, I make myself drink water.

B. Blossom Lordman

Chapter 22

Eat As Clean As You Can

When I learned portion control, it was time to change *what* I was eating. As I mentioned before, I would eat lots of fast foods, fried foods, and junk food. I changed how I cooked my food. I no longer fry anything. I bake all of my meats. I cut pork out of my diet and started eating more chicken and turkey.

I still treat myself to "bad food" from time to time, but I know when to stop now. My body knows when to stop. When I am full or satisfied, I will have my plate removed so I won't graze on the leftovers or pack it up to take it home.

I no longer sit and binge on junk food. It does not taste

the same, and it makes me feel sick. I do crave the occasional chocolate at that time of the month, but other than that, I keep my cravings under close watch.

Eating clean can be very expensive, if you let it. According to eatingwell.com, "**Eating clean** is a good way to refresh your **eating** habits: it's about **eating** more of the best and healthiest options in each of the food groups—and **eating** less of the not-so-healthy ones. That means embracing whole foods like vegetables, fruits and whole grains, plus healthy proteins and fats."

Allow me to share a few tips with you on clean eating, and how to make it a little less expensive.

1. Shop Farmers Markets for fresh produce. The prices are cheaper and the produce is fresher. I like Farmers markets because it helps our local farmers make a living, instead of helping grocery chains make a profit.

2. Ask for discounts on bruised or close-dated produce. It's nothing for me to see a bag of salad or spinach and ask the produce manager

to discount it. If I see bruised apples or any other produce, I ask the manager to mark it down. They would rather get something for it than have to dispose of it and make nothing.

3. Go for frozen produce. People tend to shy away from frozen produce. I used to as well. Frozen produce is just as good as fresh. Fruits and veggies are flash frozen as soon as they are picked. You can also ask for discounts on those as well.

4. If you can only afford canned foods, then by all means, eat them! Canned produce is not my favorite choice because they are higher in sodium, but I won't hesitate to use cans. I just rinse them off and eat them.

5. Cook produce and beans in batches and freeze them for later use. Then you know how your food is cooked and it saves trips to the grocery store.

B. Blossom Lordman

Chapter 23

Find Your Fitness

I can't begin to tell you how much I love fitness, and it all started with my beautiful sister taking me to my first spin class. I can't tell you why, all I know is my body liked it and I wanted more. I don't know if it was the music or the people, but I felt very happy being there. The name of the gym was called "The Rush," and boy was it a rush! I was mesmerized by the energy in the place and the bright lights. I was in awe of the sweaty people working out. To me it seemed like they were in their own little world. Many people had a smile on their face, and it looked as though they were enjoying their workout. I wanted to feel like that. I wanted that glow.

Somehow, I felt that this place was where I needed to be. Katrina and I started going more often, and every time I went, I wanted to go back. At first we weren't sure of what we were doing. We walked on treadmills and tried different machines.

One day we were approached by a personal trainer named Angie. I remember feeling intimidated at first when she talked to us because she was so fit! She was so nice, showing us the proper way to use the machines. I was impressed that she took the time to show us how to do things right. To this day we still remain friends.

Yes, I was in the right place! The gym offered many classes, everything from Zumba, to weight lifting. They offered Yoga and Boot Camp. Believe it or not, it was the Boot Camp class that made me truly fall in love with fitness.

Again, I was intimidated by all of the fit women surrounding me, but I had to try. This class was hardcore, and so was the instructor. I remember thinking "There is no way in hell I'm going to get through this class!" Somehow, someway, I made it, and I never stopped.

The instructor's name was Debbie, and she is the most amazing person in the world. She was hard on me. She didn't feel sorry for me, and she wouldn't let me feel sorry for myself. We did really intense exercises in her class. They were really hard for me because I was still pushing over 200 pounds, with 48DDD breasts, so running and jumping seemed impossible for me.

She had us doing everything from burpees to running the stairs with weighted balls. There were times when I thought I was either going to throw up or have a heart attack! The ladies in the class began to cheer me on. As I said before, I became friends with a good handful of the women in the class.

Debbie also introduced me to Centergy (a mix between Pilates and Yoga) and taught me the correct way to lift weights. I will be forever grateful for Debbie and the ladies in that Boot Camp class.

I also fell in love with Zumba so much that I got my license to teach! I didn't get to do too much instructing, because at that time I didn't have a car to get around, and honestly, I didn't think I was that good at it. I enjoyed the music and the dance moves. I met some really nice women in those classes as well.

My personal trainer friend also introduced me to new things. She took me on my first hike and my first bike ride. The funny thing about that bike ride is I rode great for four miles. Then I managed to get the bike back to the van and fell off. What a great time that was!

I would look for workout videos on YouTube, as well as try different workouts posted on Pinterest. You name it, I was willing to find it! Finding your fitness takes time. Try everything under the sun until you find something you like.

Chapter 24

Find a Great Support System

*T*hankfully, I found an awesome support system at the gym. I was so lucky to find people who would push me, even when I didn't want to push myself. God gave me a great group of women who wanted to help and teach me. They never judged me. They only pushed me harder.

And another thing: Don't look for everybody to be excited about your lifestyle change.

If you can't find support at home, work, or church, please don't let that deter you from your journey. Most people don't like what they don't understand, or what they are not comfortable with. People who are closest to you can be the most hurtful. You just have to brush it off and continue with your journey!

You must learn to encourage yourself as well. If you don't have self-motivation, then it is very easy to fall off of your journey. It's hard to get others to believe in you if you don't believe in yourself. Always keep in mind that your lifestyle journey is for YOU!

Chapter 25

Never Give Up

There was a time when I almost gave up. I couldn't afford to attend the gym anymore and I became very depressed about it, because I missed every single thing about the gym. I missed the music, the people. Most of all, I missed my beloved Boot Camp class. I became so depressed over the separation that I began to pick my weight back up.

I began to sneak and eat all of the foods that I had worked so hard to break free from. I stopped exercising, and I stopped caring. It didn't help that I was still a cashier at the drug store, and in my down time, I would eat junk food.

One day one of my coworkers came to me and said, "Beverly, why are letting yourself get fat again?" That was a slap in my face. Not because he called me fat, but because I was losing everything that I had worked so very hard for.

Surprisingly, I didn't cry. I didn't shout or yell at him. I simply told him the truth. I was depressed and I had to do something about it! I didn't have money for the gym, and I didn't have extra money for Zumba classes, but there had to be something else that I could do.

Luckily, this was right at the time of the year when it was beginning to warm up. One day I decided to go walking. I wasn't new to the neighborhood, but I had never ventured out on a walk. I was sort of apprehensive, but did it! I only walked for about a mile, but it was the most exhilarating feeling!

I decided to walk the next day, and the next, and the next. I loved walking! I didn't walk a trail, or a track. I walked down Wade Hampton Boulevard, one of the busiest streets in Greenville, SC. It didn't bother me that it was busy. In fact, that was one of the exciting things about it.

Even though I was no longer at the gym, I still kept in the back of my mind all of the wonderful things Debbie taught me. After walks, I would come back home and do pushups and planks. I would do those dreadful burpees, and tricep dips. With all of the walking and added strength training, I began to notice my weight drop. YES! I found my fitness again! At first I would only walk for about one mile. Today, I can walk up to seven.

B. Blossom Lordman

Chapter 26

We Walk

(Moving with Motivation)

I fell so in love with walking that I began to blog about it. I blogged more on Instagram, and to my surprise I began to have followers. I blogged less on Facebook, because I felt like I was getting on folk's nerves. Little did I know how many people were actually watching and following me there as well.

I had two other ladies who also began to sing the praises of walking. I decided to begin a support group. It was only supposed to be for ladies who loved walking. Although I was doing more than walking, I stressed walking to others because it is so easy to do.

To my surprise, this group continued to grow, in more ways than just numbers. My own story, my own journey, was really beginning to inspire and motivate others to lose weight. Not only to lose weight, but to live a healthier lifestyle.

Never in my wildest dreams would I have thought that my journey could inspire so many. Today, *We Walk* is over 1000 members and growing. Motivation is the major key in my lifestyle change.

I am thankful for this group of wonderful men and women. We keep each other accountable to work out and eat as clean as we can. I don't think I could have gotten this far without this group of amazing people.

As I inspire them, they inspire me. As I motivate them, they keep me motivated as well. No one ever said that living a healthier lifestyle was easy, but having this awesome support system makes it a lot easier.

And the Journey Continues. . .

Finally, Truly Happy

I am finally a happy woman, and it feels absolutely phenomenal. I finally have confidence in myself. My happiness no longer comes in the form of Little Debbies or Mr. Goodbar. My food addiction is something I will always struggle with, but I intend to overcome that fight.

I am happy with my job, my family, and my friends. This lifestyle change was a true lifesaver for me. Your past does not have to dictate your future. I do believe in breaking generational curses. Whether it is addiction, depression, or "family secrets," those family curses can be broken.

As I stated before, my relationship with my mother is a

hundred times better, and I know that we will only grow closer. I pray that through this book, she is cleansed as well. I don't get to talk to my sister Karen often, but I'm sure she is handling life on her own terms. I don't have the best life, but I am finally at peace with my past.

My past makes me who I am today. Do I regret some things of my past? Yes, I do. But I accept the path that God has chosen for me. I can only pray that this book will help others to open up and talk to someone about any abuse they have endured in their lifetime.

My life has been plagued with so many ugly words–molestation, abuse, and addiction. But I'm still here.

I'm here to tell the tale.

My beginning does not determine my end. I choose to live a happy, healthy life, for the REST OF MY LIFE.

More About Blossom

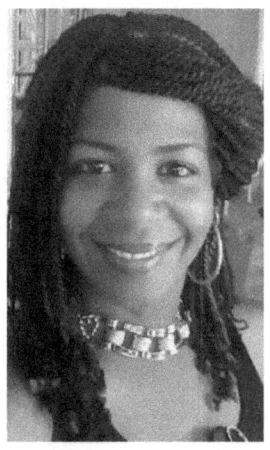

Blossom was born in raised in Asheville NC, but she resides in Greenville SC. She is a server by day at Roost Restaurant and a writer by night. Blossom is the mother of three sons and grandmother of three grandsons. Although fitness was not a part of her early life, it is her PASSION now. She enjoys sharing her journey through her social media group called *We Walk*, where she inspires and motivates others daily to live a healthier lifestyle.

Blossom plans to continue spreading the good news of living a clean and healthy lifestyle. She is available for book signings, health fairs and seminars.

Email: wewalk1@gmail.com

Website: wewalk1.weebly.com

B. Blossom Lordman